HEALTHY GUT NOW :

101 BEST FOODS FOR YOUR GUT

Health Research Staff – Millwood Media

Millwood Media

****

Published by:

Millwood Media Division

Laurenzana Press
PO Box 1220
Melrose, FL 32666 USA

LaurenzanaPress.com

HEALTH DISCLAIMER

TABLE OF CONTENTS

INTRODUCTION

Ready to embark on an exciting journey to transform your gut health? You're in the right place! This book isn't just a list of foods; it's your guide to understanding and nourishing one of the most crucial parts of your body - your gut. And trust me, your gut deserves some serious love and attention.

Why Focus on the Gut?

Let's start with a fun fact

Did you know your gut is often called the "second brain" of your body? It's true! This isn't just because it decides when you feel hungry or full; your gut health influences everything from your mood to your immune system. That's why what you feed your gut is super important.

The Superheroes of Gut Health

High-Fiber Foods

Enter high-fiber foods, the superheroes of the gut world. You might have heard people talking about fiber, and they're onto something big. Fiber isn't just good for keeping you regular (although that's a pretty nice perk). It's essential for your gut's overall health.

Two Types of Fiber

Soluble and Insoluble

Here's where it gets interesting. There are two types of fiber - soluble and insoluble. Think of soluble fiber as a sponge. It absorbs water and turns into a gel during digestion, slowing things down and helping you feel full. It's great for controlling blood sugar levels and can be found in foods like oats, apples, and beans.

Insoluble fiber, on the other hand, is the tough guy. It doesn't dissolve in water and adds bulk to your stool, which helps everything move through your digestive system more smoothly (goodbye, constipation!). You can find it in whole grains, nuts, and many vegetables.

Both types of fiber are important for a happy, healthy gut, so you want a good mix of both in your diet.

The Magic of Short Chain Fatty Acids

But wait, there's more! When you eat high-fiber foods, something amazing happens in your gut. The good bacteria there ferment the fiber, especially the soluble kind, and create something called short-chain fatty acids (SCFAs). These little fatty acids are like super fuel for your gut cells. They help keep your gut lining strong and reduce inflammation. This isn't just good for your digestive health; it also plays a role in preventing diseases like diabetes and heart disease.

They also contribute to emotional well-being by influencing neurotransmitter production, maintaining the integrity of the blood-brain barrier, and modulating the stress response.

They're some of the biggest Superstars of the gut.

More Gut-Friendly Chemicals

Besides SCFAs, your gut bacteria also produce other important chemicals when they munch on fiber. These include vitamins and other compounds that help your body function at its best. Like the feel good chemicals serotonin and dopamine. It's like your gut is a little chemical factory, producing all sorts of goodies that keep you healthy and feeling good.

The Power of a Fiber-Rich Diet

So, what does all this mean for you? A diet rich in high-fiber foods can transform your health. It can help you maintain a healthy weight, reduce the risk of chronic diseases, and even improve your mood. And the best part? These foods are delicious!

101 Best Foods for The Gut

We're going to dive into the tastiest, most gut-friendly foods out there. We're talking about fruits bursting with flavor, crunchy veggies, hearty grains, and so much more. And we're not just listing these foods; You'll get all sorts of cool tips and facts about each food. Did you know that raspberries are fiber power-houses? Or that quinoa is a complete protein?

Whether you're a cooking pro or just starting out, you'll find something here that's perfect for your kitchen

Your Companion on the Journey to Better Health

101 Best Foods for The Gut is more than just a book; it's your companion on a journey to a healthier you. By the end of it, you'll not only understand your gut better but also know how to take great care of it with every bite you take.

So, are you ready to start this adventure? Let's dive into the world of delicious, gut-friendly foods and discover how a few simple changes to your diet can make a world of difference to your health and happiness. Here's to a journey of tasty foods and a healthier, happier gut!

"DISCOVER THE FUTURE OF GUT HEALTH AND BULLET-PROOF YOUR IMMUNE SYSTEM"

Welcome to the next generation of gut wellness with our groundbreaking formula, meticulously designed for those who prioritize holistic health.

This is what makes **GUT GRUEL** your best bet for treating gut issues:

✓ **Oat Bran:** Not just another grain! Brimming with beta-glucans, this VIP super fiber may be the very best gut food around. This gut superhero ensures your digestive tract experiences smooth sailing while it helps regulate your blood sugar, improve your immunity, lower your cholesterol while it fights off inflammation.

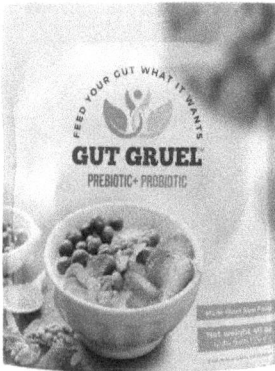

✓ **Golden Flaxseed Milled:** Beyond its glittering name, golden flaxseed offers a bounty of dietary fiber, supporting your gut's quest for regularity, while its omega-3s act as peacekeepers, keeping inflammation in check.

✓ **Inulin:** Think of this as your gut's favorite snack. This prebiotic is the unsung hero behind a thriving, balanced microbiome.

✓ **Coconut:** A tropical touch with a purpose! Its rich MCTs act as guardians, fending off harmful microbes, ensuring your gut is a sanctuary of health.

✓ **Allulose:** Light sweetness without the side effects! Experience the joy of a natural sugar alternative that keeps your gut environment undisturbed and in perfect harmony.

✓ **Cinnamon:** A dash of spice and everything nice. With its innate anti-inflammatory properties, it's the shield your gut always wished for.

✓ **Sea Salt:** Nature's own mineral mine. These crystals fortify your gut lining, ensuring it stands strong against daily challenges.

✓ **Live Active Cultures:** *Bacillus coagulans* and *Bacillus subtilis*, proven to survive the high heat and acid of the stomach, dive deep, working their magic, ensuring your gut biome thrives, flourishes, and evolves.

The journey to optimal gut health is now just a scoop away. Dive into this elixir and feel the transformation from within. Let your gut be the compass leading you to a life less ordinary. Join us in this revolution, and let's redefine wellness together!

Learn More at www.GutGruel.com

Almonds

Almonds are a superb choice for enhancing gut health, as they're not only a healthy source of fats but also rich in fiber. This combination makes almonds an excellent snack for satisfying hunger and promoting digestive wellness. Each ounce provides a substantial 4.2 grams of fiber, supporting a healthy gut microbiome. Additionally, almonds are packed with manganese, vitamin E, and magnesium, which contribute to overall well-being. Whether enjoyed in salads, trail mixes, or as a chocolate-covered treat, almonds are a versatile and gut-friendly addition to any diet.

Apples

Apples are a delicious ally for gut health, thanks to their pectin content — a type of fiber that's excellent for appetite control and promoting a healthy digestive tract. These fruits are not only sweet and satisfying but also rich in polyphenols, offering antioxidant support. With just 95 calories per medium-sized apple and 5.7 grams of fiber, they're a fantastic choice for maintaining a healthy gut. Remember to eat them with their skin on for the maximum fiber boost.

Apricots

Apricots are a small yet mighty fruit when it comes to gut health, boasting a significant amount of beta-carotene. Low in calories, with just 16 per fruit, apricots are also a great source of vitamins A and C. Diets rich in beta-carotene are linked to heart health, which is essential for overall well-being. With 3.5 grams of fiber in a four-apricot serving, they're an easy and tasty way to support your digestive system. Add them to oatmeal or whole wheat toast for a gut-friendly meal.

Artichoke

Often overshadowed by more common vegetables like broccoli, artichokes are a powerhouse for gut health. They're an excellent source of folic acid, making them ideal for pregnant women, and are also high in vitamin C, supporting immune function. With 5.4 grams of fiber per 100-gram serving, artichokes aid in stabilizing blood sugar levels and controlling hunger. They also contain antioxidants like Quercetin and gallic acid, which further enhance their health benefits.

Avocado

Avocados stand out in the fruit world due to their healthy fat content and high dietary fiber, with 13.5

grams per fruit. These attributes make avocados fantastic for heart health and reducing inflammation, which is beneficial for gut health. Studies show that diets rich in avocados can improve blood lipid concentrations more effectively than high-carb diets. Their creamy texture also makes them a versatile ingredient for various dishes.

Bananas

As a commonly eaten fruit, bananas are known for their richness in vitamin B6, C, potassium, and manganese. Ideal as an energy booster due to their high potassium content, bananas also support cardiovascular health with their 2.8 grams of fiber per serving. Additionally, they are stomach-friendly and aid in electrolyte restoration, making them great for digestive health.

Barley

Barley is a whole grain often overlooked in favor of brown rice, but it's a fantastic choice for boosting fiber intake. With 4.2 grams of fiber per half-cup, barley is beneficial for cholesterol management and intestinal health. It's also a great source of manganese and magnesium and helps reduce the risk of type 2 diabetes.

Incorporate barley into soups, casseroles, or salads for a gut-healthy diet.

Beets (cooked)

Cooked beets, with 2.8 grams of fiber per cup, are a nutritious addition to any diet. They contain betalains, phytonutrients that offer antioxidant and anti-inflammatory benefits, helping to protect against diseases. Rich in folate, manganese, and potassium, beets are excellent for overall health and particularly beneficial for eye health.

Beet Greens

As an alternative to regular lettuce, beet greens provide about 1.5 grams of fiber per cup, along with calcium, magnesium, potassium, vitamin C, and B-vitamins. These nutrients, along with additional antioxidants, help reduce the risk of diseases like cancer, making beet greens a healthy and nutritious choice for gut health.

Black Beans

Black beans are exceptional for digestive health, containing a whopping 13.9 grams of fiber per cup. High in molybdenum, they maintain normal enzyme levels and, with their mix of protein and fiber, are ideal for blood glucose control, reducing diabetes risk. They're a nutritious choice for maintaining a healthy digestive tract.

Blackberries

Blackberries are a fiber-rich berry, providing 3.8 grams per half-cup. They're abundant in antioxidants, vitamin E, folate, magnesium, potassium, and copper, offering robust immune support due to their high vitamin C content. Blackberries are a versatile fruit that can be added to oatmeal, smoothies, or yogurt, making them a great choice for gut health.

Black-Eyed Peas

High in fiber at four grams per serving, black-eyed peas are excellent for heart health and stabilizing blood glucose levels. They're rich in potassium, essential for muscle and nervous system function, and provide zinc for cellular metabolism and immune support. Don't overlook this nutrient-packed legume for your gut health.

Blueberries

For antioxidant protection, blueberries are unmatched. They help prevent free radical damage, which can lead to cancer, and are great for cardiovascular health. With 4.2 grams of fiber per cup, they're a delicious way to support gut health. Add them to yogurt or oatmeal for a healthful start to your day.

Bok Choy

Bok Choy, a versatile vegetable, contains 0.7 grams of fiber and is an excellent calcium source, aiding in osteoporosis prevention and muscle contractions. With fiber making up almost half of its carb content, it's a nutritious option for salads or stir-fries.

Brazil Nuts

Often overlooked, Brazil nuts are a nutritional powerhouse, fighting inflammation and helping control blood sugar levels due to their fat and low carb content. Each cup offers 10 grams of fiber and 19 grams of protein, along with magnesium, phosphorus, and copper.

Broccoli

A 'must-have' for health, broccoli is loaded with anti-oxidants for cancer prevention and is low in calories. With 2.4 grams of fiber and 2.6 grams of protein per cup, it supports reduced inflammation and detoxification, and is linked to lower rates of cardiovascular disease.

Brown Rice

A popular grain, brown rice has more fiber than white rice, with 1.4 grams per half-cup serving. It helps control hunger and energy levels by moderating blood sugar release. Rich in manganese, magnesium, and iron, brown rice ensures proper red blood cell development and energy levels.

Brussels Sprouts

Brussels sprouts, containing 3.6 grams of fiber per cup, offer detoxification benefits and boost the immune system. They also provide antioxidants for free radical damage protection and inflammation reduction.

Buckwheat

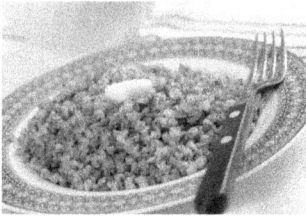

Buckwheat, a grain abundant in fiber with 8.5 grams per half cup, is an excellent choice for gut health. It's rich in manganese, aiding in blood pressure and cholesterol management. Regular consumption of buckwheat can decrease diabetes risk by ensuring better blood sugar control, making it a valuable addition to any meal plan for maintaining a healthy digestive system.

Cabbage

Cabbage, a nutrient-dense vegetable, offers just 19 calories per cup but is packed with 2 grams of fiber and a gram of protein. It provides significant cancer protection due to its antioxidant content and supplies an array of nutrients including vitamins A, C, K, B6, folate, magnesium, potassium, and manganese. As a healthy alternative to lettuce, cabbage is a gut-friendly addition to your diet.

Cantaloupe

Cantaloupe, a sweet melon, matches an orange in vitamin C content and fulfills daily vitamin A needs. It's beneficial for eye health, preventing cataracts, and lung health, reducing emphysema risks. With 1.4 grams of fiber per 53-calorie cup, it's an excellent snack for promoting gut health.

Carrots

Carrots, a popular vegetable, are an excellent source of vitamin A, providing over 600% of daily needs per cup. They are high in beta-carotene and antioxidants, supporting cardiovascular health and healthy eyesight. Each large carrot offers 2.6 grams of fiber, contributing to digestive health.

Cashews

Cashews are a diverse nut rich in copper, magnesium, and tryptophan, and high in monounsaturated fats for heart health. They help stabilize blood sugar levels and reduce diabetes risk. With 1 gram of fiber per ounce, cashews contribute positively to gut health and a balanced diet.

Cauliflower

Cauliflower, part of the cruciferous family, boosts immune support with nearly 100% of daily vitamin C in one cup. It aids in detoxification, reducing illness risks, and provides strong antioxidant support against oxidative stress. With 2.5 grams of fiber per cup, cauliflower is excellent for bowel health and blood sugar regulation.

Celery

Celery, a low-calorie vegetable at only 14 calories per chopped cup, is loaded with vitamins K, C, potassium, and folate. It provides 1.6 grams of fiber per cup, making it predominantly fiber-rich and excellent for hydration, supporting gut health and digestion.

Chestnuts

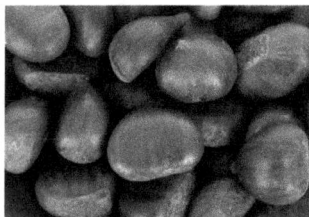

Unlike most nuts, chestnuts are lower in calories and fat but high in fiber, offering 8.1 grams per 100 grams. They are a good source of carbohydrates, folate, oleic acid, iron, calcium, potassium, magnesium, and zinc, beneficial in salads or stir-fries for digestive health.

Chickpeas

Chickpeas, a key vegetarian protein source, are rich in molybdenum, manganese, folate, tryptophan, phosphorus, and copper. They provide digestive support and reduce cardiovascular disease and diabetes risks. With 4 grams of fiber per half-cup, chickpeas are an excellent dietary addition for gut health.

Coconut

Coconut, known for its sweet flavor, is rich in medium-chain triglycerides, a heart-friendly saturated fat. It reduces heart disease risk, lowers cholesterol, improves digestive disorders, enhances thyroid function, and offers 7.2 grams of fiber per cup of shredded coconut, supporting gut health.

Collard Greens

Collard greens, excellent for cholesterol management, bind bile acids in the digestive tract. With 30 calories and 3.6 grams of dietary fiber per cup, they're rich in iron, calcium, copper, manganese, selenium, B vitamins, and vitamin K, reducing Alzheimer's risk and promoting bone health.

Corn

Corn, a popular vegetable, provides vitamin B1, folate, and vitamin C. It offers digestive support and stabilizes blood sugar levels with 1.7 grams of fiber per half-cup, contributing to a healthy gut.

Cranberries

Known for urinary tract health benefits, cranberries also provide anti-inflammatory and antioxidant support. They boost the immune system with proanthocyanidins and contain 4.4 grams of fiber per cup, aiding in gut health.

Black Currants

Black currants, rich in vitamin C, strengthen the immune system and protect against illness. They offer antioxidants to combat free radical damage and supply 6.8 grams of fiber per 100 grams, promoting digestive health.

Dates

Dates, a fast-acting carbohydrate source, contain tannins for inflammation reduction and are rich in beta-carotene and lutein. With 1.6 grams of fiber per date, they help stabilize blood sugar levels and manage cholesterol, supporting gut health.

Ezekiel Bread

Ezekiel bread, a healthy bread variety, offers 3 grams of fiber and 4 grams of protein per 80 calorie slice. Its higher fiber content helps reduce blood sugar spikes, making it a gut-friendly option for meals and snacks.

Fermented Foods

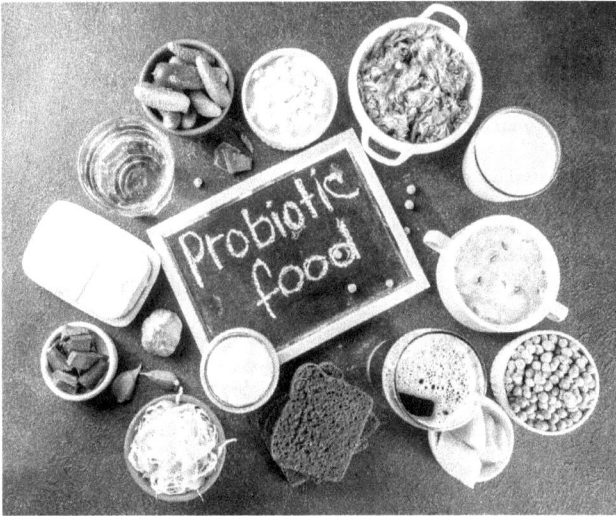

Fermented foods are culinary staples that undergo a process where natural bacteria feed on the sugar and starch in the food, creating lactic acid. This natural fermentation not only preserves these foods but also creates beneficial enzymes, B-vitamins, Omega-3 fatty acids, and various strains of probiotics.

Nutritionally, fermented foods are diverse as they include a range of products like yogurt, kefir, kombucha, sauerkraut, tempeh, and kimchi. Common to all is their probiotic richness, which is crucial for maintaining a healthy gut microbiome. These probiotics aid in digestion, help in the absorption of nutrients, and strengthen the immune system.

Regular consumption of fermented foods has been linked to improved gut health, better digestion, and even a reduced risk of certain chronic diseases. They're particularly important in a diet for promoting intestinal health and restoring the balance of bacteria in the gut.

Each fermented food has its unique nutritional profile. For example, kefir is high in protein and calcium, while sauerkraut offers a good dose of fibers and vitamins C and K. Tempeh, a fermented soy product, is a great source of protein and vitamin B12, especially beneficial for vegetarians and vegans.

Integrating fermented foods into your diet can be simple and delicious. They can be used as flavorful side dishes, like kimchi with meals, or as part of main dishes, like tempeh in stir-fries. Yogurt and kefir are excellent for breakfast or as healthy snacks. Regularly including these foods can greatly contribute to a balanced, gut-friendly diet, and offer a world of flavors and textures to explore.

Flaxseeds

Flaxseeds, rich in omega-3 fatty acids, fiber, and protein, offer 4.8 grams of fiber per 2 tbsp. serving. They reduce inflammation and prevent high blood pressure, making them a great addition to oatmeal, smoothies, or baked goods for gut health.

Figs

Figs, a high-fiber fruit with 5.3 grams per 3 fig serving, are beneficial for blood pressure management due to their potassium content. They're also calcium-rich, promoting strong bones and making them a healthy addition for active lifestyles and gut health.

Garlic

This nutrient-rich food is a boon for gut health, packed with vitamins C, B6, and compounds like allicin. It supports cardiovascular health, lowers blood pressure, and has antimicrobial properties. As a prebiotic, garlic boosts beneficial gut bacteria, aiding digestion and potentially preventing digestive cancers. Its antioxidants also combat cell damage. Easily added to various dishes, garlic enhances both flavor and health, making it a valuable part of a gut-friendly diet.

Grapefruit

Grapefruits, rich in vitamins C and A, potassium, and folate, contain just 72 calories per fruit. Their lycopene content reduces prostate cancer risk and protects against Alzheimer's. With 3.1 grams of fiber, grapefruits support gut health.

Green Beans

Green beans, with only 43 calories per cup, are rich in vitamins K, C, A, manganese, potassium, iron, and omega-3 fatty acids. They provide cardiovascular benefits and improve insulin sensitivity. With 2 grams of fiber per half-cup, green beans are a healthy vegetable for gut health.

Guava

Guava is an often overlooked fruit that's a powerhouse for gut health, offering nine grams of dietary fiber per 112 calorie serving. It's an excellent source of vitamin A, folate, potassium, copper, manganese, and especially rich in vitamin C, providing over 600% of your daily intake. This makes guava not only great for your immune system but also for maintaining a healthy digestive system.

Hazelnuts

With 2.7 grams of fiber per ounce, hazelnuts surpass Brazil nuts and cashews in fiber content, promoting healthy digestion. They contain a balance of healthy monounsaturated fats and a low amount of saturated fat, beneficial for heart health. Hazelnuts are also rich in vitamin B6, folate, arginine, vitamin K, and vitamin E, supporting overall wellness including gut health.

Honeydew

This sweet melon, honeydew, is a nourishing choice with a gram of fiber per serving and only 64 calories. It's a great source of vitamin B6, folate, potassium, and vitamin C, aiding metabolism and immune strength. Its fiber content helps in maintaining a healthy digestive system.

Kale

Kale is a nutrient-dense vegetable packed with vita-mins K, A, C, E, and essential fatty acids. With 1.3 grams of fiber per cup when cooked, it offers anti-inflammatory and antioxidant benefits, along with aiding in detoxification, which is beneficial for gut health.

Kidney Beans

Kidney beans are a fiber-rich choice with 5.8 grams per half cup, also loaded with folate, manganese, phosphorus, iron, potassium, and magnesium. These beans are great for stabilizing blood sugar levels and maintaining cognitive function, making them an excellent addition to a gut-healthy diet.

Lentils

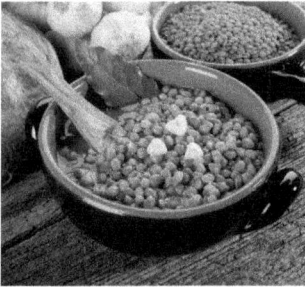

Easy to prepare, lentils provide 6.6 grams of fiber per half-cup, effectively reducing the risk of irritable bowel syndrome. Regular consumption can lower the risk of coronary heart disease and, with their high iron content, they help in maintaining consistent energy levels throughout the day.

Leeks

Leeks contain the flavonoid kaempferol, promoting blood vessel health and aiding in the relaxation of blood vessels. They also protect against oxidative stress linked to various diseases. With 1.6 grams of fiber per 54 calorie cup, leeks are great for weight management and supporting gut health.

Lima Beans

Lima beans, with 13.2 grams of fiber per cooked cup, are excellent for blood sugar control. Rich in tryptophan, manganese, folate, potassium, iron, copper, and phosphorus, they're a powerful addition to your diet for reducing heart attack risk and promoting digestive health.

Macadamia Nuts

For nut enthusiasts, macadamia nuts are a fiber-rich choice, offering 2.3 grams per ounce. They're high in heart-healthy unsaturated fats and iron, ensuring optimal red blood cell production and energy levels, making them a beneficial addition for gut health.

Mushrooms

Mushrooms are a versatile vegetable that's packed with nutrients like riboflavin, niacin, pantothenic acid, vitamin B6, thiamin, and folate. They contain almost a gram of fiber per cup and only 15 calories. High in protein content, they support metabolic function and digestive health.

Millet

Millet, a unique grain, offers a creamy yet fluffy texture and is used in couscous preparation. It's rich in magnesium, beneficial for asthma and migraine prevention, and niacin, which aids in cholesterol management. With 3.3 grams of fiber per half cup, it's a great grain for maintaining blood sugar levels and supporting gut health.

Oats

Oats are a standout breakfast choice, high in fiber and protein, and low in sugar. With four grams of fiber per cup of cooked oatmeal, they're excellent for managing cholesterol levels and providing long-lasting energy. Oats also contain beta-glucan, important for immune system enhancement and infection prevention.

Oat Bran

As an alternative to oats, oat bran offers 6 grams of protein and 7 grams of fiber in a one-cup prepared serving, with only 88 calories. Sugar-free and rich in iron, it's a satisfying choice for a healthy start to the day, particularly for gut health.

Olives

Often added to pizzas and salads, olives are a high-fiber food with 3.3 grams per 3.5 oz. serving. They contain healthy fats and unique phytonutrients like hydroxytyrosol, which help prevent cancer and bone loss. Rich in iron, they're beneficial for preventing anemia and maintaining energy levels, supporting digestive health.

Okra

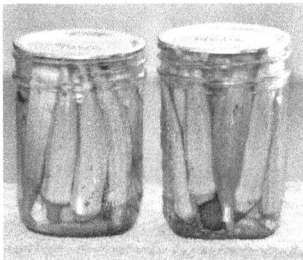

Okra, with 7 grams of dietary fiber per 10 oz. serving and only 71 calories, is an excellent addition to weight loss diets. Low in cholesterol and sodium, it provides zinc, copper, vitamins A, C, K, thiamine, riboflavin, folate, calcium, and magnesium, along with 5 grams of protein, making it an ideal food for vegetarians and gut health.

Onions

Regular consumption of onions reduces the risk of various cancers and provides chromium, which helps stabilize blood glucose levels. Rich in vitamin C, manganese, folate, and sulfur, onions promote connective tissue strength and bone health. Each cup contains 1.5 grams of fiber, making them a valuable addition for digestive wellness.

Orange

Oranges, famous for their vitamin C content, also provide thiamin, potassium, vitamin A, and a dose of calcium. Consuming oranges supports the immune system and alleviates inflammation-related conditions. With 3.4 grams of fiber per fruit, they are a convenient and healthy choice for gut health.

Papaya

Papaya, a seasonal fruit, is exceptionally high in vitamin C, providing over 300% of daily intake. Also rich in vitamins A, E, K, and folate, papaya is beneficial for colon cancer prevention and digestive health. With 118 calories per fruit and 5.5 grams of dietary fiber, it's a must-have for a healthy gut.

Passion Fruit

Often forgotten, passion fruit is a rich source of vitamin C, vital for immune strength. It also provides vitamin A, potassium, iron, copper, and magnesium. With an impressive 25 grams of fiber per cup, passion fruit is excellent for blood sugar control and digestive health.

Peaches

Peaches, a sweet treat rich in vitamin A and beta-carotene, promote good eyesight and vision. High in potassium, fluoride, and iron, they support strong teeth, bones, and healthy blood pressure levels. With 2.4 grams of fiber per peach, they are a delightful addition to a gut-healthy diet.

Peanuts

Peanuts, a popular legume, are rich in manganese, tryptophan, vitamin B3, folate, and copper. They offer a protein boost and 2.3 grams of fiber per ounce, making them excellent for gut health. Peanuts are versatile in salads, stir-fries, or snack mixes, and their niacin content has been linked to reduced Alzheimer's disease symptoms.

Peanut Butter

Peanut butter is a versatile condiment with 2 grams of fiber per 2 tbsp. serving. It provides 8 grams of protein and 16 grams of mostly unsaturated fats, aiding in blood sugar control and hunger management. Rich in niacin and manganese, it's a gut-friendly option for toast, bananas, or smoothies.

Pears

Pears, a sweet and juicy fruit, are great for hydration and provide 4 grams of fiber per serving, supporting cardiovascular and colon health. With vitamin C and a low allergy risk, they are a safe choice for those with severe allergies. Each pear adds 97 calories to your diet, making it a nutritious, gut-healthy choice.

Peas

Peas offer a wide range of nutrients, including vitamins K, C, manganese, B1, folate, A, phosphorus, and magnesium. They are beneficial in reducing inflammation-related disease symptoms and are excellent for blood sugar regulation. With 4.4 grams of fiber per half-cup, peas are a great addition to any gut-friendly diet.

Pecans

Pecans, popular especially during the holiday season, provide 2.7 grams of fiber per serving and support cholesterol and blood sugar management, and cognitive function. Rich in vitamin E and plant sterols, they have cholesterol-lowering properties and are recommended for heart health.

Peppers

All varieties of peppers, including red, green, or orange, are beneficial for immune health due to their high vitamin C content. Each cup offers 1.6 grams of fiber and is rich in vitamins A and E, along with carotenoids for antioxidant benefits. Capsaicin in red peppers has been linked to prostate cancer cell growth inhibition.

Plums

Plums are a simple, low-calorie fruit with 36 calories per serving, providing vitamins C, A, and B2. They enhance iron absorption, making them ideal when paired with iron-rich foods. With 2.2 grams of fiber per serving, plums are effective in satiating hunger.

Pinto Beans

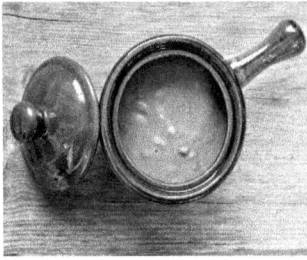

Pinto beans are high in fiber with 7.4 grams per half-cup, also offering molybdenum, folate, and manganese. They are an iron-rich option for vegetarians and can lower heart attack risk and stabilize blood sugar levels. A BMJ journal study showed a lower blood sugar response to beans compared to other carbohydrates.

Psyllium Seed Husks

Psyllium seed husks are a fiber-rich choice, providing 9 grams of fiber per two tablespoon serving, making them almost a pure fiber food. Ideal for controlling blood glucose and calming hunger, they are a great addition to shakes, oatmeal, or baked goods.

Pistachio Seeds

Pistachios are rich in oleic acid and antioxidants, maintaining healthy cholesterol levels. High in vitamin E and minerals like copper, manganese, potassium, calcium, iron, zinc, and selenium, they offer over 10 grams of fiber per 100 grams, aiding appetite control.

Popcorn

Popcorn, when prepared healthily, contains 3.5 grams of fiber per 3 cup serving and only 93 calories. It also offers 3.1 grams of protein, making it a filling snack on a lower calorie diet.

Potato

Potatoes, though often avoided for their GI index, are nutrient-packed when eaten with protein and healthy fats. Rich in vitamin C, B6, copper, and potassium, they provide 4.8 grams of fiber per medium potato, aiding in blood pressure management and cardiovascular health.

Prunes

Prunes, ideal post-workout for muscle glycogen restoration, offer vitamin A, potassium, and copper. They contain unique antioxidants for cellular protection and are high in potassium, supporting cardiovascular health. With 3.1 grams of fiber per serving, they're excellent for daily fiber intake.

Pumpernickel Bread

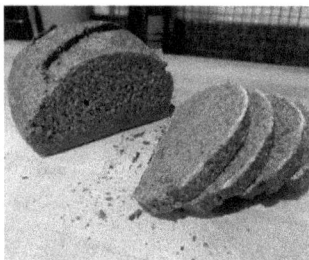

Made from rye, pumpernickel bread is a high-fiber option with 2 grams of dietary fiber per slice and only 65 calories. It's low in saturated fat and a good source of selenium and manganese.

IMPORTANT: Locally made pumpernickel bread with no additives, emulsifiers, etc is gut friendly. Most commercial pumpernickel breads don't measure up. Check your local farmer's market or co-op for quality sources – or make your own!

Pumpkin

Pumpkin, versatile in dishes beyond pie, offers unique flavors and health benefits. With 83 calories per cup and over 7 grams of fiber, it's ideal for weight management. Rich in manganese, magnesium, niacin, phosphorus, potassium, thiamin, and vitamin C, pumpkin is a nutritious choice.

Pumpkin Seeds

Pumpkin seeds, more than a Halloween treat, have a sweet and nutty flavor. Rich in manganese, magnesium, iron, and vitamin K, they contain over one gram of fiber per ounce, making them a healthful addition to salads or trail mix.

Quinoa

As a brown rice alternative, quinoa is not only fiber-rich but also a complete protein source. High in manganese and magnesium, it's beneficial for migraine relief and cardiovascular health. With 4.2 grams of fiber per half-cup cooked, quinoa is a must-have for a gut-friendly diet.

Raisins

Raisins, perfect for active lifestyles, are antioxidant-rich and help combat free radical damage. They contain boron for bone strength and offer 5.4 grams of fiber per cup. While high in calories, they're a valuable energy source in moderation.

Raspberries

Low in sugar and high in fiber, raspberries offer 6.4 grams of fiber per cup and only 60 calories. They provide significant antioxidant support, more than strawberries, and are rich in manganese, vitamin C, riboflavin, folate, niacin, magnesium, potassium, and copper, making them a great choice for any diet.

Rye Bread

Rye bread is a high-fiber alternative to regular bread, aiding in energy stability and hunger satisfaction. It helps prevent insulin resistance, reducing diabetes and metabolic syndrome X risks. With 2.7 grams of fiber per slice, rye bread is effective in controlling blood glucose responses.

IMPORTANT: Locally made rye bread with no additives, emulsifiers, etc is gut friendly. Most commercial rye breads don't measure up. Check your local farmer's market or co-op for quality sources – or make your own!

Sesame Seeds

Rich in healthy fats and providing 3.3 grams of fiber per ¼ cup, sesame seeds are a nutritious addition to your diet. Excellent for sprinkling over salads, they offer copper, magnesium, and calcium. They're particularly beneficial for those with rheumatoid arthritis due to high copper content and can help lower blood pressure, reducing heart disease and stroke risks.

Sourdough Bread

This tangy, fermented bread is great for gut health. It's rich in prebiotics, aiding beneficial gut bacteria, and packed with B vitamins. Each slice offers about 3g of protein and 2g of fiber, supporting digestion and blood sugar control. The fermentation lowers its glycemic index, making it a healthier choice over white bread. Sourdough is ideal for mild gluten sensitivities, though not for celiac disease. It's versatile, perfect for sandwiches or avocado toast, and contributes to a balanced, gut-friendly diet.

IMPORTANT: Locally made sourdough bread with no additives, emulsifiers, etc is gut friendly. Most commercial sourdough breads don't measure up. Check your local farmer's market or co-op for quality sources – or make your own!

Soybeans

Soybeans are a staple in vegetarian diets but are also excellent for anyone seeking more fiber and protein. They provide 4.9 grams of fiber per half-cup and are rich in tryptophan, manganese, iron, and essential fatty acids. Consuming soybeans can aid in lowering blood pressure and maintaining healthier cholesterol levels.

Spinach

Swap out regular lettuce for spinach in your salads for a nutrient boost. Spinach is loaded with vitamin K, A, manganese, and folate, and is vital for maintaining healthy red blood cells. With 41 calories and 4.3 grams of fiber per cup, spinach consumption can reduce the risk of cancer, particularly prostate and breast cancer.

Split Peas

Low in fat and high in protein and dietary fiber, split peas offer a substantial 16.3 grams of fiber per cup. They are also high in potassium, essential for muscle contractions, and are low in sodium, making them ideal for blood pressure management.

Strawberries

At only 43 calories per cup, strawberries are a sweet, fiber-rich berry, offering 4.4 grams of fiber per serving. They're loaded with vitamin C, manganese, iodine, potassium, and folate, and contain B vitamins. Strawberries, packed with antioxidants, have been shown to inhibit carcinogenesis and modulate inflammatory processes.

Summer Squash

Packed with manganese, vitamin C, magnesium, vitamin A, and other nutrients, summer squash is excellent
for blood sugar control and offers anti-inflammatory
benefits. With 2.5 grams of fiber per ½ cup, it's a valuable addition to any diet.

Sunflower Seeds

A convenient snack, sunflower seeds are rich in vitamin E, beneficial for asthma, osteoarthritis, and
rheumatoid arthritis, and contain phytosterols to lower cholesterol. With over 7 grams of fiber per half-cup,
they aid in nerve function, muscle contraction, and
vascular health.

Sweet Potato

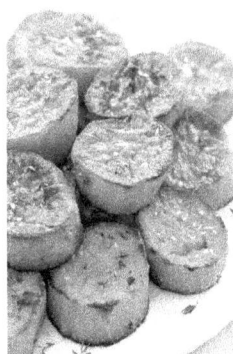

A better choice for blood sugar
management than regular potatoes, sweet potatoes are lower on
the GI index and rich in vitamin A,
manganese, copper, and offer 4.9
grams of fiber per medium potato.
Try them as cinnamon-sprinkled
fries for a healthy snack.

Swiss Chard

Rich in vitamins K, A, C, magnesium, and potassium, Swiss chard is especially beneficial for those with diabetes, aiding in blood sugar control. With almost 3.5 grams of fiber per cooked cup, it's a nutritious alternative to lettuce in salads.

Tomatoes

Tomatoes, high in lycopene, are excellent for prostate and colon health. They're also rich in vitamins C, A, K, potassium, manganese, and B vitamins. Each tomato provides 1.3 grams of fiber, contributing to a well-rounded nutritional intake.

Turnip Greens

Often overlooked, turnip greens are a nutrient-dense food, providing vitamin K, A, C, folate, manganese, and calcium, with just 28 calories per cup and 1.8 grams of fiber, making them an easy fit in any diet.

Turnip

Low in calories with just 17 per half cup and offering 1.6 grams of dietary fiber, turnips are a rich source of folate, calcium, potassium, copper, manganese, vita-min C, and B vitamins, ensuring prolonged satiety.

Walnuts

Rich in essential fatty acids, walnuts are not only deli-cious but also a powerhouse for gut health. Each one-ounce serving boasts 3.1 grams of dietary fiber, crucial for maintaining a healthy digestive system and pre-venting inflammatory diseases like metabolic syn-drome, cardiovascular disease, and type 2 diabetes. Additionally, walnuts are abundant in manganese, copper, and tryptophan, offering a spectrum of essen-tial nutrients vital for overall wellness and gut health.

Winter Squash

Distinguished by its unique flavor, winter squash is a nutritious choice, particularly high in vitamin A. The starches in winter squash are beneficial for stabilizing blood glucose levels and maintaining healthy insulin levels, important factors in gut health. Although low in fat, it provides a valuable source of omega-3 fats, often lacking in diets. With 3.1 grams of fiber per half-cup serving, winter squash is an excellent addition to your diet for promoting digestive health.

Wheat Germ

Wheat germ is an effortless way to increase your fiber intake, essential for gut health. Providing four grams of fiber and six grams of protein per ounce, it's an ideal addition to any meal. Easily incorporated into oatmeal, muffins, or pancakes, wheat germ enhances your digestive wellness with its high fiber content, playing a key role in a healthy gut.

Wheat Bran

Starting your day with wheat bran contributes significantly to gut health. High in Thiamin, Riboflavin, Potassium, fiber, Niacin, vitamin B6, iron, magnesium, zinc, and copper, it's a nutritional powerhouse. With only two grams of fat per cup but 24.8 grams of dietary fiber and 9 grams of protein, wheat bran is a superb choice for maintaining a healthy digestive system.

White Beans

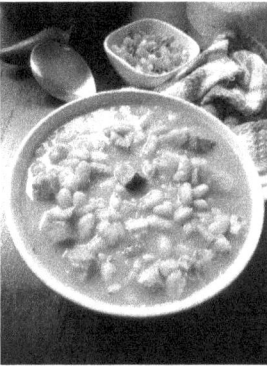

White beans, with 11.3 grams of fiber per cup and minimal sugar, are excellent for steady blood sugar levels and gut health. Low in sodium and cholesterol-free, they're an ideal protein source for vegetarians and beneficial in maintaining healthy cholesterol levels, thereby supporting heart and digestive health.

Wholegrain Pasta

For those leading active lifestyles, whole grain pasta is a superb energy source, thanks to its rich complex carbohydrate content. Besides providing energy, it also offers a moderate amount of protein and 5 grams of fiber per serving, making it a great choice for supporting digestive health.

Yams

Yams are an excellent alternative to regular potatoes, especially for those concerned with blood sugar levels. With a lower GI index and packed with 8.9 grams of dietary fiber per medium yam, they're ideal for appetite control and gut health. Baked with cinnamon,

they make a delicious treat that also supports digestive wellness.

Yeast (Bakers)

Incorporating bakers yeast into your baked goods is
another way to enhance fiber intake, crucial for a
healthy gut. It's a high source of iron, preventing iron-
deficiency anemia, and rich in protein, Thiamin, Riboflavin, Niacin, Vitamin B6, Folate, and Pantothenic
Acid. With one gram of fiber per 18 calorie serving,
it's beneficial for appetite control and digestive health.

Zucchini

Zucchini, a fantastic vegetable for hunger management, is loaded with Niacin, phosphorus, copper, vitamin C, Riboflavin, Vitamin B6, folate, magnesium,
potassium, and manganese. At just 20 calories per
cup, it's weight-loss friendly and excellent for regulat-
ing blood sugar levels, thus maintaining steady energy and supporting gut health.

CONCLUSION

So there you have some of the top foods for your gut that you should be adding to your diet on a regular basis. Diversity is the key to good gut health. Diverse bacteria and diverse food (AKA fiber and resistant starch) for that bacteria.

Aim to add as many fermented foods as you can to your diet to get more diversity of bacteria. Try to eat 20-30 foods in this book every month to keep the bacteria happy and working for you. That adds the diversity of food that they love.

Remember to always add more fiber to your diet in moderate amounts to increase your body's comfort level with upping your dosage. If you go too quickly and add 20-30 extra grams of fiber per day, you're very likely to experience gastro-intestinal distress, cramping, bloating, excessive gas, and possibly even diarrhea.

It is normal to experience gas when consuming fiber. That's the by-product of the bacteria fermenting the fiber, so that's a good thing. It means your gut is working! When it becomes too excessive for you, dial back your fiber intake a bit and hold there for a while before gradually adding more.

These recommended daily amounts of fiber should be considered your MINIMUM.

Men under 50 years are recommended to have 38 grams per day.

Men over 50 years are recommended to have 30 grams per day.

Women under 50 years are recommended to have 25 grams per day.

Women over 50 years are recommended to have 21 grams per day.

IMPORTANT: Always remember that fiber absorbs water, so when you increase your fiber intake, it's important to also increase your water intake to help the fiber move through the digestive system. Adequate hydration can help prevent the constipation that sometimes accompanies higher fiber consumption.

HANDY LIST FOR SHOPPING FOR THE 101 BEST FOODS FOR YOUR GUT

Below you will find the foods listed in a section where you might find them in a grocery store. Some items may be found in more than one place in your store so that is why you will find them listed in more than one section below. Whenever possible … eat FRESH … not canned or preserved. When you must choose canned or frozen, read ingredients to make sure no additives are included. Enjoy!

FRESH FRUITS and VEGETABLES

Apples

Apricots

Artichoke

Avocado

Bananas

Beet greens

Beets, cooked

Blackberries

Blueberries

Bok Choy

Broccoli

Brussels sprouts

Cabbage

Cantaloupe

Carrot

Cauliflower

Celery

Collard greens

Corn

Cranberries

Figs

Grapefruit

Green beans

Guava

Honeydew

Kale

Leeks

Mushrooms

Okra

Onions

Orange

Passion fruit

Peaches

Pears

Peas

Peppers

Plum

Potato

Pumpkin

Raspberries

Spinach

Split peas

Strawberries

Summer squash

Sweet potato

Swiss chard

Tomato

Turnip

Turnip greens

Winter squash

Yam

Zucchini

BAKING AISLE

Coconut

Currants

Dates

Yeast, bakers

CEREAL/RICE /PASTA AISLES

Barley

Brown rice

Buckwheat

Oat bran

Oats

Wheat bran

Wheat germ

Wholegrain pasta

CONDIMENTS

Olives

DRIED LENTILS/CANNED VEGETABLES

Black beans

Black-eyed peas

Chickpeas

Kidney beans

Lentils

Lima beans

Pinto beans

White beans

FROZEN FOOD SECTION

Broccoli

Brussels sprouts

Carrot

Cauliflower

Corn

Cranberries

Green beans

Okra

Onions

Peaches

Peas

Spinach

Strawberries

Sweet potato

NUTS/DRIED FRUIT SECTION

Almonds

Brazil nuts

Cashews

Chestnuts

Hazelnuts

Macadamia nuts

Peanuts

Pecans

Pistachio seeds

Popcorn

Prunes

Pumpkin seeds

Raisins

Sesame seeds

Sunflower seeds

Walnuts

HEALTH FOOD SECTION or HEALTH FOOD STORE

Brown rice

Buckwheat

Flaxseeds

Millet

Oat bran

Oats

Peanut butter

Psyllium seed husks

Quinoa

Soybeans

Wheat bran

Wheat germ

FROZEN HEALTH FOOD SECTION

Ezekiel bread

FARMER'S MARKET/FOOD CO-OP

Pumpernickel bread

Rye bread

Sourdough bread

Many of fresh fruits and
vegetables on the list

REFERENCES

Barker, H.M. et al. (1980). Exceptionally low blood glucose response to dried beans comparisons with other carbohydrate foods. BMJ Journal. 281:578. August 30.

Binkoski, Amy. Et al. (2009). The Effects of Nuts On Coronary Heart Disease Risk. Nutrition Reviews. Vol. 59, Issue 4, pp. 103-11.

Branca, F. (2003). Dietary Phyto-oestrogens and bone health. Proceedings of the Nutrition Society. 62, 877-887.

Burke, K. et al. (2001). A monounsaturated fatty acid-rich pecan-enriched diet favourably alters the serum lipid profile of healthy men and women. The Journal of Nutrition. 131:2275-2279.

Colquhoun, DM. et al. (1992). Comparison of the effects on lipoproteins and apolipoproteins of a diet high in monounsaturated fatty acids, enriched with avocado, and a high-carbohydrate diet. The American Journal of Clinical Nutrition. Vol. 56, pp. 671-67.

Desmond, J. C. et al. (2006). Capsaicin, a component of red peppers, inhibits the growth of androgen-independent, P53 mutant prostate cancer cells. Cancer Research. 66(6) 3222-9.

Giordano, C. et al. (1986). Low glycemic response to traditionally processed wheat and rye products bulgur and pumpernickel bread. American Journal of Clinical Nutrition. Vol., 43, 516-520.

Giovannucci, E. et al. (2002). A Prospective Study of Tomato Products, Lycopene, and Prostate Cancer Risk. Journal of the National Cancer Institute. Vol. 94, Issue, 5. Pp. 391-398.

Greenberg, E.R. (1997). Intake of carrots, spinach, and supplements containing vitamin A in relation to risk of breast cancer. Cancer Epidemiology, Biomarkers & Prevention. 6; 887.

Hannum, Sandra. (2004). Potential Impact of Strawberries on Human Health
A Review of the Science. Critical Reviews in Food Science and Nutrition. Vol. 44, No. 1.

USDA FoodData Central
https://fdc.nal.usda.gov/fdc-app.html

WHICH OF THESE CONDITIONS DO YOU HAVE?

- **Tummy Troubles:** Feels like your stomach is always upset, with cramps, gas, bloating, or a sense of being overly full.
- **Running to the Bathroom:** Either you're constantly constipated, feeling like you're carrying bricks in your belly, or it's non-stop diarrhea, like your insides are in a rush to get out.
- **Tired for No Reason:** Even after a good night's sleep, you feel like you're dragging through the day, like your body's batteries are always low.
- **Acid Reflux (GERD):** You're often tasting a sour, acidic backlash, a reminder that your stomach is not keeping its contents to itself.
- **Craving Junk Food:** You can't seem to get enough of sugars and carbs, almost like your body's addicted to the bad stuff.
- **Mood Swings:** You're up one minute, down the next, feeling like you're on an emotional rollercoaster.

- **Headache Haze:** Frequent headaches or migraines that make your head feel foggy or like it's in a vice.
- **Skin Issues:** Breakouts, rashes, or itchy skin that make you feel like you're having a never-ending bad skin day.
- **Joint Pain:** Achy joints, like you're older than your years, making moving around feel like a chore.
- **Catching Colds Easily:** You catch every bug going around, feeling like your immune system is on a permanent vacation.
- **Food Intolerance:** Suddenly, some foods just don't agree with you, leaving you feeling sick or uncomfortable after meals.

Take the FREE Gut Health Quiz and Find Out More

www.LaurenzanaPress.com/101Best

###

www.ingramcontent.com/pod-product-compliance
Lightning Source LLC
Chambersburg PA
CBHW060634280326
41933CB00012B/2038